Operation D-Rek

Operation D-Rek

By

Derek Canas

Copyright © 2018 by Derek Canas

All rights reserved. This book or any portion thereof may not be reproduced or used in any manner whatsoever without the express written permission of the publisher except for the use of brief quotations in a book review.

Printed in the United States of America

First Printing, 2018

ISBN 978-1719017688

Table of Contents

Dedication	iii
Introduction	iv
Chapter One: A Brief History of HIV/AIDS	1
What are HIV and AIDS?	
HIV/AIDS Epidemic	
Chapter Two: Preliminary Medical Issues	6
Open-Heart Surgery	
The Surgery & Recovery Tim	
Notable Moments	
Chapter Three: Medical Issues Between Initial Surgeries and the Age of 16	15
My Childhood	
Life as a Big Brother	
Summers with Grandma	
Favorite Memories	
School, Medical Stuff, and Struggles	
Chapter Four: HIV Diagnosis and the Aftermath	31
Growth Hormones	
The Possibility of HIV	
The Day of the Diagnosis	
Aftermath	
Family Reaction	
The Stigma	
Unexpected Complications	
A New Normal	
Feeling a Little *Too* Good	
DJ D-REK	
Chapter Five: Various Medical Mishaps	65

PSA: End the Stigma!	75
My Campaign	78
Conclusion	83

Dedication

This book is dedicated to my family. You've stood beside me as I've been tossed through life. Thanks for always being there to keep me laughing. I know it's not easy to stand beside a hospital bed and you've done it every time for me. You've watched me pull out I.V.s, on accident of course, and snuck food inside the hospital and even snuck me out. You've helped with meds and post op care.

I owe my family everything they are the reason I get back up out of the hospital. Here's to the doctors both good and bad you've given me one great story to tell, and to the Grim reaper you missed me again asshole. I wrote this book to show that strength and courage come in all shapes and sizes. This is a lesson on survival through laughter.

Introduction

I'm writing this book to not only share my story, but also to encourage everyone reading to take some time to really understand what HIV/AIDS is, how it is contracted, and the myths surrounding it.

I want us to work together to end the stigma and to spread awareness and understanding, and that's not something we can do unless we're all on the same page. While you're reading my story, I hope you're able to see that I'm just a normal guy despite my struggles. Throughout everything, I've just kept moving forward and lived my life.

Thanks for reading, and please take a moment to look up my campaign to end the stigma once and for all!

Chapter One: A Brief History of HIV/AIDS

In the relatively few decades that I have been alive, society has changed a great deal. Conditions that were considered lethal 30 years ago have often been studied extensively and rendered, at the very least, *less* lethal than they once were. Unfortunately, this has the side effect of essentially muting the discussion regarding the syndromes and diseases in question. This can lead individuals to have a false sense of security that encourages reckless or uninformed behavior – behavior that could lead to significant health complications.

What are HIV and AIDS?

One of the most well-known viruses in the world is that of HIV. Also known as the human immunodeficiency virus, HIV is a condition that leads the body to break down its own immune system. As a result, patients have trouble warding off things like diseases and infections and can eventually lead to the development of acquired immunodeficiency syndrome, or AIDS. AIDS is known as the most severe and serious phase of the HIV virus and infection. It can lead to patients running into more and more opportunistic infections, including certain forms of cancer. There is no known cure for HIV or AIDS, however when caught early and treated effectively, it is possible to treat HIV. Modern medicine has dramatically improved the prognosis of these individuals over the years. Note, however, that the virus will never leave the body fully – when someone is diagnosed, they will have the infection for life.

HIV/AIDS Epidemic

In the 1980s and the 1990s, HIV/AIDS were among the feared and misunderstood health issues in the world. It is no exaggeration to say that there was a full-blown HIV/AIDS epidemic during this point in time, especially in the United States. The virus and resulting infection claimed the lives of thousands of individuals during this time and was often transmitted between partners via sexual contact. One huge issue during this era was that the virus and subsequent infection were poorly understood by the medical community. There was even a widespread misconception that HIV/AIDS were only an issue in the LGBTQ community during that time, leading many individuals to believe that they were "safe" as long as they didn't engage in homosexual sexual contact. Today, of course, we know that this is not the case. While the virus *was* more common in the gay community than among other populations during the 1980s and 1990s, it had little to do with the form of sexual contact in question.

Because HIV/AIDS was so poorly understood, it is perhaps not surprising that the virus was unintentionally transmitted even in hospitals. Today, we know that things like blood transfusions can lead to the development of the HIV virus in individuals who receive a transfusion of infected or tainted blood. Unfortunately, this knowledge wouldn't become more publicly known until the mid-1980s, leading thousands of individuals to contract HIV after receiving a blood transfusion for an entirely unrelated incident. Hospitals wouldn't start widespread screening of their blood supply for the virus until 1985, and even then, it took years for the screening to be perfected and universally adopted. Even infants receiving blood transfusions during something like a surgery were at risk for contracting the virus.

How do I know? Well, I was one of those infants. In 1985, at just three months old, I underwent open heart surgery and received a blood transfusion. And although I wouldn't become aware of this for sixteen more years, the blood that I received was tainted with HIV.

Chapter Two: Preliminary Medical Issues

You might wonder why I went into the history of HIV/AIDS in the United States. Well, the answer is a simple one: I wanted you to better understand the circumstances I was facing when I had my first surgery at the age of three months old. With that background, what ultimately happened to me might not make immediate sense. As we get into the beginning of my story, I just want you to keep in mind that this all began in 1985, the very same year that hospitals in the United States received permission to use new commercial tests to screen for HIV in their donated blood supply.

Unfortunately, the HIV virus was incredibly misunderstood during this time, and it would be another few years yet before the medical community at large and the general public had a better idea about how exactly the virus spreads. That also means that the urgency of screening donated blood had yet to set in – while the risk of infection via blood transfusion was acknowledged during 1985, it wasn't yet recognized that the risk of infection could be fairly great. In fact, many blood banks and hospitals at this point still believed that the chance of infection via blood transfusions would be "very low" – somewhere within one individual per one million patients transfused, according to a joint statement released by the Council of Community Blood Centers, the American Association of Blood Banks, and the American Red Cross in 1983.

Well, those numbers might not be far off – not today, at least, when blood screening has become the standard. But between the years of 1981 – the first reported case of HIV in the States – and 2001, an estimated 14,260 individuals were diagnosed with HIV resulting from blood transfusions (this is according to a study conducted in 2003)[1]. In a single decade, in other words, well over 14,000 individuals in the United States contracted HIV via a transfusion. These numbers rapidly increased during the 1980s and peaked during the 1990s[2].

Why am I so focused on these numbers and the timeline? Well, I had surgery in 1985. I received no less than 15 blood transfusions during my

---

[1] Donegan, E. (2003). Transmission of HIV by Blood, Blood Products, Tissue Transplantation, and Artificial Insemination. Retrieved fromhttp://hivinsite.ucsf.edu/InSite?page=kb-07-02-09

[2] CDC (2001). "HIV and AIDS - United States, 1981--2000." MMWR (Website). Retrieved from https://www.cdc.gov/mmwr/preview/mmwrhtml/mm5021a2.htm

stay in the hospital – and I am one of the more than 14,000 individuals who contracted HIV via a transfusion.

Open-Heart Surgery

I was three months old when I had open-heart surgery for the first time. If that sounds serious, that's because it was, and even more so when you remember that this took place over thirty years ago and medical advancements were not quite what they are today. The problem that led to my surgery was first detected during my three-month checkup. My parents opted to take me to see a new pediatrician, and during the visit my lips began to turn blue as I cried. That is when it was first suspected by a medical professional that I had a heart issue, and it was here that my heart murmur was detected for the first time.

I saw another doctor the next day in Jacksonville, Florida, who did their own examination. They determined that I had transposition of great arteries in my heart, and I was sent to Augusta to undergo open-heart surgery.

The Surgery & Recovery Time

The surgery itself was not an easy one. It took the majority of the day to complete, and I would not come out of it unscathed (in many ways). The surgeons disrupted my heart rhythm during the procedure, for example, and I had to have a pacemaker installed in order to help regulate my heartbeat. Additionally, I received several pints of blood throughout the operation, as well as afterwards.

I suppose that the surgery was more or less considered a success at the time, despite the necessity of installing a pacemaker in my heart to help my heart beat normally. With that said, it should not be assumed that the process was an easy one. Today, the process of repairing transposition of the great arteries in infants is often described as a surgery that necessitates a few-day stay in an ICU ward followed by a few more days elsewhere in the hospital once discharged from ICU. The entire process, from surgery to discharge, generally takes between two to three weeks. When I had my surgery in 1985, I was in the ICU for three months after surgery was completed. I spent much of that time on machines designed to help my body breath and my heart to beat.

During the recovery period in the ICU, I struggled with a number of side effects. My kidneys almost shut down, I had seemingly unending fevers and infections – I even had fluid buildup in my lungs that necessitated the use of chest tubes. As you might imagine, throughout all of this I was in need of many blood transfusions. Multiple members of my family volunteered to donate blood to me for the procedure. The hospital turned these requests down, stating that this wasn't "hospital policy" and that my family should calm down – the blood came from their blood bank, and everything would be okay. With no other choice, my family trusted the medical professionals that assured them the process was a safe one and focused on seeing me through my surgery and subsequent recovery.

By now, we all know that the blood transfusions I received weren't an "everything will be okay" situation. On the contrary, they were the source of my HIV infection. Before we continue examining the medical issues that plagued me after this first surgery, however, I'd like to take some to talk about how my hospital stay affected my family members as well members of the hospital staff.

Notable Moments

One very notable event that always sticks out in my mind when I think about my time in the hospital as an infant is that of my mother's sleeping arrangements. My family had a room at the local Ronald McDonald house, but my mom rarely went there. She slept on a waiting room floor outside the ICU room most nights, wanting to be as close to me as possible.

There was a nurse in the ICU who, every day before she left, would always stop by to say goodbye to me. Before she would leave, she always asked me to smile for her. Note that at this point, I was in the ICU, chest tubes, surgery scars, and should have been miserable – but I smiled at her every single time. I spent three months in intensive care, but thankfully I learned a new skill - I learned to flirt.

   Another moment relayed to me by my family members over the years that always sticks out to me is one that occurred between my grandfather and my nurse. My grandfather, whom I would eventually name Pop-Pop, a retired marine and an instructor for the capital police, FLETC in Brunswick, GA, was visiting me in the hospital when he noticed a nurse trying to force feed me. I wasn't doing too well with how she was trying to feed me, and he ultimately kicked her out of the room and found the head nurse on the floor and told her that we wanted a new nurse and stood guard until they brought another nurse. He was also there for my first night out of the ICU! It was a was guys' night, just me and him. My grandfather was there giving some other family break for a little while, and he called my mom and my grandmother and said, "you'll never guess who I'm hanging out with in a private room."

Chapter Three: Medical Issues Between Initial Surgeries and the Age of 16

My surgery at three months old was not the only medical issue I would deal with throughout my youth. Some of the main medical issues that I dealt with after the initial surgery were mostly bronchitis and pneumonia as well as the fact that I wasn't growing at the pace that I should have been due to the virus that was, at that point, hidden. Its presence caused many, many health problems that we'll talk about in a later chapter. For now, suffice to say that I dealt with medical issues throughout my childhood and the vast majority of them stemmed from the HIV virus that I was unknowingly fighting.

With all of that said, I don't want to spend the entirety of this book just recounting my medical struggles. After all, humans can persevere under even the most horrible of conditions – and while I wouldn't say that I had a particularly "healthy" childhood (in the strictest sense of the word), I did have a very fun childhood. From playing with other kids on the playground to doing embarrassing things in public, I'd say that my youth was pretty great. I want to share some of my history with you guys. Maybe the stories will help you get a better sense of who I am.

My Childhood

My entrance into the world was not calm and quiet like a "normal" life would appear. The way I entered the world was my mom was in Maryland for my uncle's birthday.

So, this entire day I'm hearing about balloons, cake, and all kinds of great things for a big party - and I wasn't invited! Well, as my mom decided that she was about to make the cake, I decided it was time to break out a month early. So, I became what you could call the ultimate party crasher. I surprised and shocked my family in a big way that day, but now I have a birthday buddy every year and that's really cool. I love that.

Everything about my life has pretty much, since that moment, been crazy, chaotic, fun, and nonstop in laughter. We just roll with what happens. That's all I know how to do, honestly, and it's an attitude that has served me well so far.

My childhood was very fun and, I'd say, fairly normal. I didn't have too many major problems outside of a couple hospital stays. And even with the hospital stays, I'd get some antibiotics and bounce right back pretty fast. I didn't let much get in my way, I guess you could say, and it seemed like my family and I always found a way to have fun.

Heck, even as a baby I knew how to have fun and make everyone laugh! My Nanny and Pop-Pop will tell you a story that happened when I was about 9 or 10 months old. I was at their house, and I don't know who had decided to change my diaper, but I had recently started crawling and I'd escaped from whoever it was and proceeded to crawl down the hallway. And at some point during the process, somebody grabbed a camera took a picture of my bare butt crawling towards freedom.

Well, after that they got me, put the diaper on me, and then dropped the film off to be developed. Weeks after the fact - you know, things weren't developed instantly back then - they were looking at the pictures and they noticed that I had peed in the hallway as I was crawling, and it went unnoticed until the picture was developed and brought back home! And yes, my grandmother still has that picture. I'm probably going to have to pay a lot of money to make sure it stays hidden in her house somewhere. But that's OK.

Another example of the fun I had as a kid would be my first vacation with my mom and dad as an example. We went down to Orlando, Florida, and then on to Daytona and went to Sea World. At the time my mom was pregnant with my little sister and was still running around with me and having a blast. My mom and dad and I spent a lot of time on the beach, and my dad is a daredevil and loves the ocean. He bought this little yellow raft and took me out on it. We make it way out past the breakers, pretty much with the full intention of giving my mom a heart attack. She somehow didn't have one despite watching her baby boy drift further and further into the water, thankfully, and we all survived. That began the start of my daredevil career in life. Now I love the ocean and going out.

Now at the end of that trip happened what is probably my Nanny's favorite story to tell people about me. When I got back from vacation, she asked me how it went. And I told her the biggest thing I remembered was that my dad took "the wrong 'effing' turn!" This was at three years old and I did *not* use the slightly politer term I just wrote above – no, I went full force into the mother of all curse words.

To be fair to my dad, driving in Daytona is confusing and there are a lot of one-way streets. I've done it recently and I, too, have taken the wrong turns! Thankfully, I didn't have a three-year-old in the back seat to tell on me, but it happens. It's very easy to happen down there and it's just one of those things.

Life as a Big Brother

When I was three years old, I became a big brother. Like many older siblings, I wasn't too sure about her at first! My Nanny likes to tell the story of the time I was supposed to go to meet my baby sister and was appalled at the thought of my mom being in a hospital with another baby. That did not sit well with me at all! That didn't last long, though, and I became my sister's protective big brother pretty quickly.

One funny story happens when I was probably five years old. My mom took me and my sister to see the doctor, and it was time to get our shots. Well, I got my shot and I was okay with it - but nobody was leaving the room. I knew something was up. I ended up getting pulled out of the room while they gave my little sister a shot, and she started crying. Well, I stormed back in the room and basically yelled at everybody and told them that I knew that was going to happen and that I was *not* very happy about it! I was always trying to be the guardian for her, even though I was about two feet tall at the time. I guess you never really think you're as small as you are.

Summers with Grandma

Here's a fun memory from the other side of the family with my Granny and Grandpa. They run a family business - a telephone repair business. And all throughout my young years my granny kept me, my sister, and my cousin Morgan through most of the summers growing up - so from the years of five, six, seven, eight, nine, all the way through about twelve years old. We were always with her. She's a very, very brave woman for doing this, by the way. Keeping all three of our little minion butts had to have been a headache, but she did well with us.

She would even take us in stores, which is still amazing to me because I know us... and I would never have been that brave.

And she always was outside with us. Granny played kickball, hide and go seek, she helped us basically destroy her house and kept us fed like we were kings.

You can never get better service in life than to spend time with your grandparents.

Favorite Memories

Some of my favorite memories will always be fishing with my grandfather and my cousin, Morgan. My grandfather still has the original fishing poles that he bought me and my cousin over 30 years ago, which I think is really cool.

In addition to the above, there are a few more favorite memories that I'd like to share with you. One of them is the time that me and my cousin, Morgan, decided to lip-sync to Kriss Kross' *Jump* in the local mall. Now, there is video evidence of this somewhere, but believe me when I tell you that I pray it stays buried in someone's closet! We look hilarious - we even dressed up just like Kriss Kross.

Another moment I want to share is one that my mom actually remembers far better than I do. When I was ten years old, I had to have my first pacemaker replacement. Well, I was with my family and my doctors getting ready for the surgery, and they gave me the relaxing "happy juice" right before they took me back to the surgical area.

Well, I decided it would be a great idea - at 10 years old - to sing a song to the nurse. And my choice was Alan Jackson's *I Don't Even Know Your Name*. I sang this song all the way down the hall until the doors shut and my family could no longer see me. Everyone in the surgical team was cracking up.

A very big part of my life has always been video games. Even when I was three years old, I knew how to set up the Nintendo - and this was back in the days where you had to jump behind a TV, switch off RF boxes, and be on the right channels and deal with cartridges that never worked. I learned how to troubleshoot technology from a very, very early age.

When my sister came along, life became even more fun because somebody else was there to be Player Two now, and she still to this day loves video games. She has kicked many of her boyfriends' butts over the years in video games, and then these guys realize "oh, you grew up with a brother. That's why you're so good."

Poor Amber, after years of being Player Two, she finally became a better player than me and my cousin Morgan. When Nintendo 64 came out, it changed the world and changed our lives. There was a game called Super Smash Brothers and my sister was really, really good at it. She would destroy us every time! I hated playing that game if my sister was around because you just couldn't beat her - she was too good.

When I was ten years old, a big family vacation happened and my Granny and Grandpa, my Aunt Debby, Uncle Mark, Mom, Dad, Amber, Morgan, and my cousin Hannah, all decided to pack up and go to Daytona Beach for, I believe, a week. We had a big condo, and everybody stayed in one spot and had a blast. One time, we bought a bunch of yellow rafts and all of us tried to give our moms heart attacks. My dad kept me out on the water pretty deep, and that not only gave my mom a near heart attack but also gave *his mom* a near a heart attack as they both watched their kids and grandkids cracking up and going way deeper than we probably ever should have in a little yellow raft right off the beach.

Also, on that trip, we made a little side trip to Orlando, Florida, to the coolest theme park you can go to on the East Coast: Universal Studios. This is one of the greatest memories to me because we had so much fun there and it was all of us kids' first time being introduced to these crazy theme park rides... rides that are not even there now, but we still talk about how terrifying it was to go and how we screamed on Jaws the first time we saw the shark come out of the water and attack the boat.

I mean, there are so many good memories from that trip and plenty of good pictures hiding around, too. I can't wait to go back and look now.

School, Medical Stuff, and Struggles

As far as school is concerned, I had a rather normal and uneventful childhood. I went to a private Catholic school from kindergarten to seventh grade. I was always very smart - always on the honor roll - and kept up very well in a classroom. The playground was a slightly different story, although I did pretty well holding my own.

The first memory I have regarding my health happens when I was probably five or six years old. I remember calling my scar a zipper because the scar from the initial surgery goes from my collar bone all the way down my sternum to my belly button, just like the zipper on a jacket. Like I said, we always managed to have fun regardless of what I was facing.

Moments where I struggled will always be trying to keep up with other kids. Due to having the heart problems and the pacemaker, I didn't have the stamina to keep up and play all day. That was always, and still to this day, is a struggle. I'd also say that I knew I was different from other kids very early on, just from the amount of time spent going back and forth to hospitals. I didn't see that happening with other family members or classmates. I knew from very early on that I was different.

I did spend a lot of time consulting different medical professionals as I grew up. I saw a cardiologist every few months for the first few years of my life, and then it went to every six months. I saw the same doctors the whole time. I was followed by the same medical team for 15 years.

I want to leave you one last story – a story that I think sums up the overall theme of my life. Now, I was – and am – the entertainer of the family. My mom tells me that when I was two years old, I knew how to turn the stereo on and would dance and entertain and keep everyone laughing. When my little sister came on the scene, it got even more fun. We had a blast singing and dancing!

It was a happy childhood. There were more smiles than tears, and that's been true throughout this entire tale.

Chapter Four: HIV Diagnosis and the Aftermath

Remember, the diagnosis of HIV was all brought about by the surgery to install a pacemaker. The operation for the pacemaker replacement went well, however I had a very hard time coming out of anesthesia. I had a hard time catching my breath. Additionally, I had a cough before surgery. I was cleared by my doctor and all of the cardiologists who would be involved in the surgery, however, to move forward. But the cough didn't go away after the operation ended.

After the pacemaker procedure, I was very sick once I got home. I was waking up at night completely unable to catch my breath. I went to see my pediatrician several times, and he diagnosed me with having asthma. All he was giving me was inhalers, and they didn't help at all. A friend of my mom's, Bobbi Mealling, helped her get me in to see a pulmonologist, Dr. Levy. When he met me, he immediately knew that there was something wrong – that there had to be more wrong than what was on my charts. He explained to me that my heart had nothing to do with my height or weight.

Growth Hormones

The doctor started running more tests to determine why I was so small and what was causing my illness. He originally thought that I had cystic fibrosis, however those tests came back negative or inconclusive. That's when an appointment was made in Gainesville for me to go see an endocrinologist. It was an intern there that ultimately suggested an HIV test when, after six months of the growth hormones, I was not growing at the rate that they had hoped.

You see, the growth hormone was a last-ditch effort for me to gain a bit more height and weight. It worked a little bit, but nowhere near as much as it should have. This led to more questions and more tests, which, in turn, led to the suggestion of an HIV test.

The Possibility of HIV

This was, as you can probably imagine, an incredibly difficult time for me. I had many questions about how, if it wasn't my heart interrupting my health, height, and weight, then what was it? Thoughts just ran wild and rampant, and I went through every kind of crazy, potential scenario you can think of.

The very last scenario that any of us – myself and my family – would have thought about would have been HIV. It was just a huge shock when that was even brought up at all.

I spent a lot of time facing a lot of questions, and this was very chaotic and trying time in my life. I learned a lot and met a lot of great new doctors, but it's not the way you want to ever meet somebody.

My family had their own reactions to this potentially new diagnosis. We were all in shock and in disbelief that HIV was even being brought up because of the amount of surgeries and doctors that I had seen… there were so many moments where it could have been caught if that's what it was – but it wasn't caught. We were all incredulous. Nobody's mind wanted to go there because… I mean, I'd been tested for everything. How can you go through sixteen years with multiple doctors, multiple hospital stays, and multiple blood draws for different reasons and no one ever catches something as important as HIV?

The Day of the Diagnosis

When the original question of an HIV test was brought up, I submitted to the test and went home for two weeks while waiting for the call to come in and to hear the results. When that call was made, they asked us to bring extra family members to the meeting, so I had my parents, my grandmother on my mom's side, and both grandparents on my dad's side with me. I kind of knew it wasn't going to be good news that day just based on the request to bring extra family. That's never a good sign. But I was not prepared, at all, to hear HIV. I was expecting to hear something more along the lines of "the test came back negative" and that more testing was going to be needed to figure out what was wrong.

When I finally got the news, I was the last one to be told. I guess they prepared my family and then brought me in last. I walked in the room and saw my mom and dad sitting there with tears in their eyes. I didn't have to really be told. I remember the people around me talking and I guess that's what they were saying, but in my memory, it all sounded pretty much like background noise – I wasn't paying attention to that. I was more focused on the fact that my mom and dad were so upset.

After that, I just turned off mentally. I didn't want to deal with anyone, I didn't want to be touched, I didn't want to hug, smile, or laugh… everything became numb. I had never experienced anything like that before in my life. My only experience with HIV and anything like that at that point was from a show I had seen years before - Nick News on Nickelodeon. They had one special that was all about HIV and AIDs, and it had Magic Johnson and a bunch of kids that were diagnosed and living with it. I remembered watching that, and that was my only knowledge of the virus at that point.

That day also began a very educational period of my life where I sat down and would go through and read everything I could find on HIV/AIDS. The diagnosis affected me big time. Being the age, I was, I was just figuring out who I was and what I wanted to be in the world… and then everything that I thought I was just shattered in one moment. It was very devastating news in a very dark spot in my mind, with very bad ideas and just being very confrontational and angry. All the bad things that nobody would ever want to see became very prevalent for a little while, until I was able to get myself in a mindset where I was better off to combat and fight the virus.

Aftermath

Right after initial diagnosis, I went home in a complete fog. I remained that way for the next two weeks as a medical team was being put together to help me. They had never seen a case where somebody had lived 16 years undiagnosed. The medical issues that occurred because of that, outside of HIV such as dental issues, I have a curve in my spine, etc., were caused by the virus running rampant for so long. My family just tried to keep me distracted for the most part.

I didn't know at this point who my doctor would be, who I would be seeing every day in the hospital – I was just lost. I mean, I wasn't new to hospital stays or medical procedures. I think we've already established that I'm pretty much an expert at them by now, and I'd say that the same held true at age 16. But what I *wasn't* an expert with was specifically HIV/AIDS. I'd spent my life dealing with my heart issues and was an old hand at them by the time I turned 16. I was entering entirely new territory with my HIV treatment and diagnosis.

When I returned to the hospital two weeks after that initial diagnosis, I met the doctor who would ultimately save my life, John W. Sleasman, MD. The first thing he said to me was that I was going to go to his funeral; he wasn't going to go to mine. I'll be honest, that was great to hear, and it really did give me some hope that I could keep on fighting and living my life. But I also knew what I was up against.

During that same conversation, for example, I found out that almost everything – my lowly stature, my curved spine, my dental problems; all of it – tracked back to the HIV being left untreated and ultimately developing into AIDs. I was just at a complete loss… even the medical terms themselves were alien to me. T cell counts? CD4 counts? Viral loads? That day was a blur – it was just so much to keep up with. But I somehow managed to do so, and I ended the day going home with an armful of books and pamphlets and new prescriptions. Everything, at that point, became something new.

To put it simply, I embarked on a whole new challenge and a whole new task.

Family Reaction

My family was shocked – I mean, we all were. There were signs that pointed towards something other than a heart problem for years, but nobody ever thought it would go to where it went. So, everybody was just devastated and none of us had any idea what was coming next. With the heart issues, we knew what to expect. I knew how the surgeries went and how I'd feel after them.

Well, I sat down and read like crazy. I read everything I could about HIV/AIDS, about treatments, about all of it. I wanted to know my new enemy as best I could. My family's way of coping was basically to keep me occupied. They kept me out of the house and kept me busy with dinners and movies – anything fun that we could find to do, is what we did for the two weeks after diagnosis. Then treatment began, and I slowly began to come back and fight what had been an unknown enemy, so we just did our best to make some fun memories before that began. That turned out to be something easier said than done.

The Stigma

As I've mentioned above, nothing really changed with family and grandparents and cousins after the diagnosis. Everybody did their best to maintain normalcy even though nothing about life after I was diagnosed was actually normal. We all did our best to try to keep everything as close to normal as we could. We tried to maintain normal patterns and fun times and going out and having a good time as a family.

The only thing that really changed, sadly, was that when we would go out I would hear rumblings and murmurings throughout the restaurants and public spaces about me. I lived in a small town, and word of my diagnosis spread quickly - and, unfortunately, there is a lot of stigma surrounding this disease. There are a lot that people aren't educated about it.

So, going to restaurants and different things, I would hear those whispers. Nothing was ever said directly to me, but you could just tell from the glances and the mumbles exactly who the topic of conversation was. You almost always know when someone is talking about you. And this happened a couple of times in town. It doesn't happen much anymore because, since I've started the "End the Stigma" campaign, I've stood up and really tried to be a voice for the people in this community that live with the virus… the people who are still hidden due to the stigma. They're afraid to lose family and lose their jobs.

Since I've stood up and become that voice, all those mumblings and grumblings went away. We'll talk about that in further detail just a little later on in the chapter.

Unexpected Complications

Before I left the doctor the day of my diagnosis, I was warned that as the viral load - the amount of the virus in my blood – would drop due to the medication, there would be hidden viruses that would ultimately come out. These were viruses that I had already been living with but wasn't aware of because they had to compete with the HIV… and the HIV won. My attention, and my body's attention, was focused on the main problem and everything else just fell by the wayside. Until I started taking the medication, of course.

I was diagnosed in April, and about five months later, on September 10th, 2001, I spent my first day in the hospital in Gainesville, FL, to fight pneumonia. My first night in the hospital, I was not happy to be there. I'm a Georgia Bulldawg fan stuck in Gator country. I was upset and angry with life… until I realized that I was in a college town and all the nurses were pretty close to my age. They were maybe five to six years older than me, and we had a lot in common and a lot of fun conversations.

My first night in the hospital at the University of Florida in Gainesville, I checked in and I had my mom and my grandmother with me. This young nurse came in and was getting ready to start an IV. She said, "I'm actually training somebody, do you mind if I let her put your IV in?" Of course, that wasn't a problem. Then this even younger girl, probably only three or four years older than I was, came in and started inserting the IV.

Now, I want to make it clear that I have really good veins. So, I'm sitting there chatting with the girl, joking around, and I'm not paying attention to what she's doing until I hear something pop. The needle had split the vein! The young nurse gets freaked out and pulls the needle out, and blood starts rushing down my arm. She hands me towels and I've soaked through two of them before I realize the reason why there was so much blood was because there was still a tourniquet around my arm. So, I tore that off with my teeth and got her to hand me a bunch of gauze pads and held them in place while they wrapped me up.

That's how my stay at the University of Florida began! From there, it was crazy trying to laugh and stay positive while dealing with a doctor who was running me through test after test to figure out where I was on different lines of health. Every number on my blood work was telling them I should be dead, so they were very curious to get as many tests in that first day as possible.

And they did - they kept me going pretty much every day from sun-up to sun-down. I was somewhere in that hospital having some kind of testing done. I didn't get much time in my own room by myself very often.

The next morning, I awoke very early - as you tend to do in a hospital - and I turned the TV on. If I remind you of the date, September 11, 2001, at this point, I'm sure you can imagine what I saw. I was one of the older patients on the pediatric floor at that point, and I turned on the news… and subsequently watched as the second plane hit the Twin Towers in New York. I was sitting there, my world still in chaos and hectic and crazy, and ended up watching the entire world devolve into something equally as crazy and hectic.

Everybody at the hospital was just lost that day. I had every nurse and doctor on that floor in my room because I was watching the news, and most of the other rooms weren't. They would come in and check on me and check on the news all throughout that day – for most of that week, to be honest. It was just an incredibly hectic and unpredictable time in my life. In addition to experiencing the tragedy along with everyone else, I was also having spinal taps and just about every test you could think of. It was just a very, very chaotic time that - looking back on – it's still unbelievable to me. I will say, though, that that day actually bonded me very well with my entire medical team. And that was good, because I would be seeing a lot of them.

A New Normal

My new reality was very different from anything that I had ever been through with cardiology with my heart problems. The HIV was monitored on a far bigger scale and far more often.

That first year, I traveled down to Gainesville every month and had 16 to 18 tubes of blood drawn - they were checking for everything. And every month the virus was going down more and more, my immune system was starting to rebound (as it was just decimated when they initially diagnosed me).

As the virus died off, my immune system started coming back. It was just incredible to see. It's very strange to know that everything about you can be on the brink of death and still come back - but you have to put in the time and effort. For me, that meant spending a lot of time in the hospital and taking a lot of medication. I took 22 pills a day at 7, 11, 3, and 11. I will never forget those times because they made up my everyday routine. I split those 22 pills among those four times, every single day.

And it all paid off. As not fun as it was, it all paid off because I've got the virus to an undetectable level now and I've built my immune system back up. I'm as healthy as I can ever be thanks to the medication and the doctors.

I was also being followed by a new cardiology team in Gainesville. It made it easy that both teams were right down the hall from each other and that they were so close. They knew each other very well and communicated often and well. Everything was a lot easier once I transferred to Gainesville with regard to managing both health issues. Thankfully, I didn't have any cardiac issues in those first few years with the HIV treatment.

Feeling a Little *Too* Good

Fast-forward a few years to age 25, and I had a cardiology

appointment. My Nanny and Pop-Pop went with me because it was just three hours away from home and it's always nice to have someone keep you company. So, I went in for a checkup with my cardiologist, and I go into the triage area where they put the pulse monitor on my finger. I wasn't really paying attention - these nurses have known me for a while now, and we're sitting and talking and laughing. One nurse looked up at the machine and said, "this one has been acting up all day - I'll go get another."

She grabbed another and put it on my finger. It beeped as it finished its calculations. The nurse looked at it and said, "Give me a minute, I'll be back." She came back with a stethoscope and a blood pressure cuff and took my pulse manually. I was immediately run into a room and told to lay down.

I was wondering what was going on at that point - no one was talking to me, they were just telling me to relax and wait for the doctor. I was sitting in the room and playing on my phone when my cardiologist walked in. He said, "You don't listen at all, do you?" I replied "Well, not usually - but what's going on this time?" He asked me how I was feeling, and I responded that I felt fine.

In fact, I had been feeling great the week before. I was working out, running more, and getting more exercise than I ever had in my life. I was even sleeping better! He said, well, that's the issue. I asked him what he was talking about, and the nurse came over, grabbed my hand, and put it on my chest. I felt a *boom... boom... boom.* She asked me if that seemed normal to me, and I said that it seemed slow, but that it was still beating so what was the problem?

That's when I was told that my heart rate was at 36 beats a minute. Apparently, my pacemaker battery had died. It had been checked less than six months before, but apparently the battery reading was incorrect. It was time for a new pacemaker. I had killed one and had no clue.

The reason I was feeling so well was because I had never known what life was like without my heart being at least partially controlled and regulated by a machine. When the pacemaker died, and that regulation was no longer in place, of course I felt better. But they advised me that I couldn't live like that for long because the human heart can only take in so much blood at a time, and mine was overworking itself by expanding too much and bringing too much blood in. They had to get me a new pacemaker.

The best part of this story is the fact that my mom wasn't there, so I had to call her and explain to her that I had a dead pacemaker. That did not go over well… and then it *really* didn't go over well when I told her that I'd be home later that day – that they needed about two weeks to get surgery scheduled! That did not go well at all. So, for the next two weeks while I was at home, I slept on the couch in the living room and my mom would get up multiple times throughout the night to check that I was still breathing and still alive. I mean, I was assured by my doctors, who also assured all family members, that I would be fine and that while the situation was urgent, it wasn't "rush to the O.R." kind of urgent.

But, of course, no mom ever wants to hear that any kind of cardiac issues are happening to their child, and that they're coming home without them fixed.

Well, surgery day finally arrived to get the new pacemaker. Thankfully,

I was able to have the surgery in Jacksonville. That was only about an hour away from home, and it made everything a lot easier for my family. I got to meet two new cardiologists there. When I have surgery, you see, I have two cardiologists and two full medical teams that go into surgery with me.

I have to have one just for my specific heart problem and one that is for the pacemaker and its separate issues. That particular day, I was going to be undergoing seven different procedures. It was going to be a very long day. They were going to do a heart cath, send a scope down my throat, take out the old pacemaker in my stomach and implant a new one in my shoulder, and there were a few other procedures that I can't remember. I just know that I signed off on a veritable scroll of release forms before they took me into the O.R.

I was originally supposed to be back in surgery for about three hours, and I believe I was actually gone for about seven to seven and a half. My mom told me that she thought they had lost me somewhere in the hospital because they weren't getting hourly updates like they were supposed to.

Once the day and all of the procedures were done and I was back in the room, I was immediately ready to go home because it was "just" a pacemaker replacement in my mind. But I was told, very quickly, that it was way more than that and that I had to stay in the hospital a few days despite surviving all of the procedures. They couldn't just send me home. So, I begrudgingly sat around and healed for a few days, and then was able to make my way back home.

DJ D-REK

Part of the reason I wanted to leave the hospital so quickly was because I was anxious to get back to work. I believe the surgery was on a Tuesday, and at this point in my life, I was DJing on Fridays and Saturdays at a nightclub. I had a regular residency and I didn't want to miss my night. So, I was very anxious to get out of the hospital. I believe I got out on Thursday, and that Friday night I called my boss - the owner of the club - and said, "I'm fine, I'm good, I'm ready to go - let's get back to work!"

He wasn't too thrilled to say yes, to be honest, but at this point in my life I was packing the club and would always have a line of over 100 people outside waiting to get in. And everybody, hearing that I was back and had new batteries, was ready to go. I showed up to work that night with my left arm in a sling, but I was alright and fine to work. The club was quickly packed, and I got a little cocky and took the sling off of my arm, and just started moving like I normally would.

I heard an audible pop – I had just popped a stitch out of my shoulder. I had to quickly run to the bathroom and re-bandage and re-tape myself before returning to finish the night. Once you take out that incident, it was a very successful night. I've earned the name D-REK for a reason - I'm pretty hard to break.

You might be wondering how exactly I ended up working as a DJ, and to be honest I have to say I attribute some of my success to the HIV. Let me explain!

I made great friendships and met a lot of great people through some very rough moments related to the virus and my medical care, so I can't totally dislike the virus. It has led to such great friendships and relationships with doctors and people all over the world. It's very cliché to say that everything happens for a reason, but as I look back upon my life, that really does seem to ring true.

One major thing that changed as a direct result of the diagnosis was my willingness to take risks. I used to be very afraid to make decisions in life. After the diagnosis, I really wasn't. That's how I really became a DJ. I started going out with friends and socializing a little more.

Eventually, when I was a bit older and started going into clubs, I met the DJs and they started telling me and showing me what DJing was all about. This was when everything was just beginning to go digital, and they weren't quite as computer-savvy as I was. That's really how I became a DJ - through my computer skills and the fact that I went out to a very popular little spot that had karaoke.

You see, I was always very scared and timid to try actually singing at karaoke, but one night I finally picked a song - shocking the friend I was with - put it on and sang along. It's probably one of the most well-known karaoke songs out there that gets everyone singing along.

Any guesses?

It was *Ice Ice Baby* by Vanilla Ice.

Now, most people would stand in one spot and sing their song. But luckily for me, the club had just gotten wireless microphones. And when I had the opportunity to get up and sing, I was able to move around the club. This was right when camera phones were just gaining popularity, and everyone went nuts. They took pictures and videos and started singing alone. The next weekend, I got a phone call from the owner of a club who wasn't there the first night I had done it, and he said that the club was packed and that everyone was looking for me to sing and help with the music.

And that's how I really started my DJ career. I was just being a goofball and being the center of attention. It was just a little hobby, and then it moved to me having my own night, to my own weekend, and then traveling around. From there, I launched my End the Stigma campaign and D-REK's Warriors and Angels.

It is crazy to look back on and think of all of the little moments and little things that have ultimately become what I am today. When I look back at the difference between 16 years old, after just receiving the diagnosis, and 26, I'm completely different. At 16, I was completely broken apart and didn't know what I was going to be, what direction my life would take, or even how long I was going to be here. I was just moving day-by-day and had no plan or goals. It was strictly a "take it as it comes" existence.

At 26, I was an established DJ. I had changed all of the little rumblings that used to happen whenever I used to walk in somewhere. They all went away, and now nobody would even think of saying those things. I had successfully tricked the town into seeing an AIDs patient as something different. People went from whispering about me and my diagnosis with AIDs to talking about how great a DJ I was and how much they enjoyed my work. And, I hope, gave people struggling in similar situations some kind of faith – something to hold onto.

End the Stigma

The change from the person I was at 16 is a turn around that I'm very proud of. I took the success of D-REK and, at age 30, decided to use that clout and influence and start the End the Stigma campaign. So far, it has gone very well.

In 2016, I was recognized as one of the top 100 AIDs activists in the southeast. My story is getting a lot of attention, and I think that's because it's a true survival tale in every aspect. I was continually tossed through different medical situations, but always fought my way back from them and created some kind of victory for myself.

I hope people see that and realize that they are a lot stronger than they give themselves credit for. And sometimes you have to get knocked down in order to get mad enough to back up and prove, to yourself as well as others, that you can do it. You ARE great. You can be greater than anything that is in a medical chart. Those are just words - they do not define you or put your life on a specific track.

Find a goal, set it, and live for something. Go after it! That's all I did from when I was 16 to when I started DJing around the age of 22. I got an idea in my mind and just worked for it. It took time, it was slow going from that and the persistence and the non-stop working towards it, I became one of the most well-known DJs in the town. I travelled from Brunswick to Orlando and Savannah DJing. That's something I'm very proud of, and something that really is a big accomplishment.

But my biggest accomplishment is and will always be the End the Stigma campaign. I've received messages from people all over the world of support and thanks. You never know who is watching you and what impact your story could have, so I always encourage people to share their tale and get involved with different organizations and groups. All of these things help you and motivate you and move you forward.

Don't stop.

That's the entire theme of my life - just don't stop. Keep on going, move forward. You can accomplish so much more than you think you can. A little bit of progress every day leads to a huge amount of progress in six months or a year. You have to look at it that way. Every day, try to accomplish one thing. In 30 days, you could accomplish a very big goal.

It's not so much about having the time as it is *taking* the time.

Chapter Five: Various Medical Mishaps

I have a few tales that don't quite fit in with everything else, but that are pretty entertaining. I'm going to go ahead and talk about them here.

After the fourth pacemaker was implanted, about six months to a year later, I fell into a very bad atrial flutter rhythm, which basically means that the top half of my heart would decide that it was going to run a marathon, but the bottom half wasn't notified. That obviously had to be corrected to get the entire heart in sync. So, I was back in Jacksonville to have the procedure to have that corrected. And as I mentioned earlier, right after I had this pacemaker installed, I popped one of the stitches DJing.

    As I'm in pre-op getting hooked up to all of the machines, the cardiologist looks at me and comments that my shoulder didn't heal right. Well, I'm no fool, so of course I replied that it sure was weird and I didn't know what had happened there. He said that it looked like a stitch hadn't held right, which I then responded to with an innocent "oh yeah? I'm not sure how that happened." He didn't say anything more about it, but it made me laugh a bit thinking about the real reason behind the botched stitch.

    Things became rapidly less amusing at this particular procedure, however, because it ended up being quite the ordeal. They were going to correct the erratic heart rhythm by going through the pacemaker, right? And as they're about to knock me out,

I see another big machine rolled in along with two huge sticker pads placed on my chest - one on the side and one smack-dab in the middle. Did I mention they had tin foil inside of those stickers?

I immediately knew what Plan B would be if they were unable to go through the pacemaker, but it's possible that I didn't entirely comprehend what exactly that would mean for me. So, a nurse came in and knocked me out - told me I'd wake up in about an hour and that there was nothing to worry about.

I woke up seven hours later to that same nurse who was a bit frustrated with me. We had had fun in pre-op, and she teased me that I "*would* wait until she's about to get off work to finally wake up!" I started to laugh in response, when I suddenly realized that I was in the worst pain I think that I've ever been in in my life. My teeth hurt -

everything hurt. My chest was extremely sore, and when I pulled the gown up, I saw the burn marks on my check.

I quickly surmised that going through the pacemaker had not, in fact, worked and the defibrillator (Plan B) ended up being carried out. I'm glad I was knocked out for that.

The next medical emergency happened not long after the tale above. It all started with my desire to get in better shape. My dad had some free weights lying around the house, and for about two weeks I used them and did well. I stayed on the low weights and went slow, doing what I could without hurting myself and staying within the five-to-ten-pound barbell range.

Then… then, I got dumb. I saw some results, and my mind immediately reasoned that if low weight gave me small results, then big weight should give be bigger results. So, I picked up a 30-pound barbell and did a full set on my right arm. Everything was cool! I picked it up with my left arm, and immediately felt a little bit of pain. I still finished the set, of course, and went about my day. I wasn't worried about it and felt pretty good. I just didn't opt for that heavy weight again. No harm, no foul, right?

Over the next two months, I realized that I was in some pretty steady discomfort. It wasn't major pain, but there was definitely something going on. I also started to see the beginnings of what would eventually become a softball-sized knot appear on my side, and it was black and blue. I finally showed my parents, who immediately called my doctor. I was back in Gainesville with my main doctor (who, I might add, was *not* amused by this turn of events). They did some tests and couldn't figure out what was going on, so I was scheduled for surgery first thing in the morning.

I went into surgery, and I ended up being in there for around two hours. I came out and realized that I was wrapped up from the middle of my back to the center of my chest. I was all taped and covered with gauze, and I just wasn't sure why. The doctor came in and explained that I had torn muscle off of my ribcage. He said that it looked like an animal had come and just ripped it right off. The black and blue that I saw was an infection that has been caused from the bleeding of that tear, and that it tracked all the way up to my chest wall.

My body was getting ready to try and push it out, but because it had gone to my chest wall, it was destroying the tissue as it sat there. If it had broken through the chest wall, the infection would have hit my heart and killed me almost immediately. Now, normally when a doctor tells you that, you panic. I'd been through so much in my life already that I was just sort of complacent with the explanation.

What did shock me, however, was the news that my chest was now stuffed full of three feet of gauze. And that gauze? Well, it needed to be changed daily.

This is the only time my mom has ever thrown her hands up in the air and said "I'm out! I can't do it! I'm not going to be able to help you on this one." So that's one hilarious outcome - it took me almost 30 years, but I eventually found something so gross and terrible that my mom had to bow out.

The next morning after surgery was the first time the gauze had to be changed, and my mom wasn't there. She had stayed at a hotel nearby the hospital. Two doctors came in to change the bandages, and I didn't know what to expect. I'd never been through that. So, they took the bandages off to get to the gauze, and they started to pull it out bit by bit. As they're doing this, I was very quickly learning how to walk using my butt cheeks. I made it all the way to the top of the bed! The doctor asked me when I last had the pain meds, and I replied that I hadn't had them - they were the first people who had been in to see me that morning.

    They immediately stopped. They knew how painful the procedure was, and that it shouldn't be done without pain meds. One of the doctors walked over and grabbed a towel that he soaked in cold water for me, and the only thing I could do was to bite on it and bear my way through it. And that's what I did! That was my first experience with changing the gauze. The poor doctor immediately ran down the hallway, grabbed my pain meds, brought them to me, and apologized profusely. There was a mix up somewhere and they never got to me on time.

But then I was just sent home, and that's what I had to do every day. Thankfully, my Nanny had always had aspirations in her life of being a nurse - and here was her chance to shine! I couldn't do it myself because of the angle of what I would have to be doing. You can't work on your own chest - it just doesn't work. So, every day I went to my grandparents' house and I had a marine and a beautician as my doctor and nurse. And we got through it! I figured out when to take a pain pill and when to get over to their place, and we just soldiered through it.

I want to say that this was a daily activity for two to two and a half months. To this day, my doctors still can't believe that I wasn't in excruciating pain with that - but

I've just been through so much pain that my tolerance is extremely high. I break things and don't even realize it until a doctor tells me so.

There's no easy way to explain a lot of the chaos that's happened in my life other than the fact that I just don't register pain like normal people do. I don't gauge it the same. The one-to-ten pain scale doesn't, and never will, work for me. My doctor will tell you that I am one of the best at creating new pain norms for myself, which is both good and extremely bad… because if the doctor doesn't know I'm in pain, he can't help me.

PSA: End the Stigma!

HIV/AIDS is not a new disease. You can check out Chapter One for more information, but it's been a "known entity" since the early 1980s at least - that's almost forty years! Why is it, then, that the attitudes surrounding it seem to be permanently stuck in the 1990s?

No one wants to have a conversation about HIV because it's not a comfortable topic to discuss. I get it. But that doesn't mean that I agree with it, and it sure doesn't mean that the best course of action is simply to stop talking. On the contrary, I think it's important to understand exactly what HIV/AIDS is and what it means to have the virus.

We can't just ignore things that aren't comfortable for us to hear about… that's how you end up with a large portion of the world without a clear understanding of what, exactly,

HIV/AIDS is, how you contract it, and what symptoms to look out for.

My PSA is to encourage everyone to get tested and to know their own status - to be their own best health advocate. Don't rely on anyone else to look out for your safety in situations where HIV could be contracted. Also, I'd like to encourage you to just take a moment and look up the signs and symptoms on your phone. Look up how HIV/AIDS is contracted and how it's not, and all of the myths surrounding it. You can do this almost instantaneously on your phone!

We're talking about a 30+ year old disease that is still very much stigmatized and misunderstood, not only in this country, but all over the world. It's very sad and disheartening to me that it is that way. But until we can start an honest discussion about it, we will never end the stigma.

That's my PSA. Learn about HIV/AIDS and protect yourself. The more we work together, the easier it is to end the stigma.

My Campaign

I started my campaign as I turned 30 as something new - a new adventure, if you will. My 20s had been all about DJing, and I wanted to move on to something different… something that allowed me to reach out to, and educate, different communities about HIV/AIDS. It's been fairly successful!

I do a lot of online advocacy, I have a website, and do a lot with Facebook and Twitter. I also have local fundraisers sometimes for things like toy drives for local pediatric wards. My Angels and Warriors and I work together to spread awareness and knowledge about the virus in an attempt to end the stigma.

I've gone out and done multiple speaking engagements at local colleges. Sometimes I speak on a panel and sometimes I go into classrooms and speak directly to a class full of college students. It's really interesting to see the reactions when people that have seen me as a DJ walk into a classroom and all of the sudden, I'm talking about a topic that they never would have expected. It's really a great way to start a conversation when it comes to HIV and AIDs because it's clear to see, even today, that it's not a conversation that's being had.

My story has been featured in multiple magazines and news articles, not only locally but also nationally. The response that I've received has been really encouraging, from not only people who have simply read the story but also the other advocates across the country and across the world. They encourage me to keep going out and telling those stories.

The campaign means a lot to me. It is the main thing that tells me that I've grown up, finally. I spent 10 years creating a DJ legacy, something that I am personally very proud of, but I needed to do something more that my family could be proud of... something that could actually change the world. I realized how unique my story was, and that it could actually be a very beneficial one to the HIV/AIDS advocacy community.

The support that I've received as I continue to fight to end the stigma surrounding HIV/AIDS has been incredible. I've gotten messages from London, Kenya, South Africa - from all over the world - since the website launched. The campaign is growing daily at a pace that is far beyond anything I could have imagined.

It's something I'm just very proud of. It's something I can look back on and know that it will continue long after I'm gone - it's something that can be carried on by others. That, in itself, is what the campaign was built for. It was meant to start a discussion and to serve as a springboard for a discussion that is uncomfortable and not fun to have.

That's also why I wrote this book. I wanted to get my story out there, sure, but mostly I wanted to try and move one step closer to ending the stigma. I hope that I've been able to tell the story and the rough moments in a way that reminds people that it's just life - it's funny, it's sad, it hurts, it's painful, but at the end of the day you have to keep going.

Maybe that's one of the things I hope people remember most when they think about this book and look at my campaign - that this is just life. It might not be something that seems normal to everyone, but to me, it's all I've experienced. And you know what? I've learned that you just have to keep moving regardless of the diagnosis. HIV/AIDS doesn't have to rule your future, nor should it impact how others view you.

We're all just trying to live our lives as best we can, and to keep moving forward.

Conclusion

Writing this book really forced me to hold a mirror up to myself and take a good, long look at my life. It made me remember and relive moments that I had forgotten about, and I'm still in shock that all of that actually happened! When everything is all written out together, it's all very shocking and incredible, even to me.

I want to share what I consider to be the most important piece of advice that I can give with you: *there is no fate, only what we make for ourselves.* Yes, I took that from the *Terminator* series – but I feel like that's fitting! And it's so true. Just because you're in a bad situation or dealing with health issues, doesn't mean that your fate has been determined. Nothing is written already. It's up to you to decide what happens next.

"Next" is always a personal decision. Sometimes that gets lost in medical situations and in difficult life situations, but "next" is always up to us. It's up to you to set your path and what you want and where you want to go. There is no fate, only what we make for ourselves.

I also want to share the importance of setting goals, which is something I will always emphasize. Whether it is something big or something small and trivial, a goal gives you something to look forward to. Looking to the future and looking outside of yourself is something that I think is very important.

It's very easy to draw in and get lost in the darkness that can occur when you have different medical issues that you deal with day to day. It's important to find things outside of that and use them as motivation to get through the next week, next month, next six months, next year, etc. It doesn't matter whether it's a big goal or a little goal like waiting on movie to come out. All that matters is that you have something to fight for.

Just remember to keep fighting.

www.ingramcontent.com/pod-product-compliance
Lightning Source LLC
Chambersburg PA
CBHW052332220526
45472CB00001B/391